THE 10 HABITS OF

HIGHLY POSITIVE

PEOPLE

YOUR GUIDE TO A HEALTHY MIND AND BODY

BY IAN J. HUNT

Table of Contents

The information herein is offered for informational purposes solely, and is universal as so. The presentation of the information is without contract or any type of guarantee assurance.

The trademarks that are used are without any consent, and the publication of the trademark is without permission or backing by the trademark owner. All trademarks and brands within this book are for clarifying purposes only and are the owned by the owners themselves, not affiliated with this document.

Introduction

It is our habits that define who we are. The way we think, the way we perceive our world and the direction that we put ourselves in depends entirely on the habits that are a part of our lives. So, if that is the power our habits have in shaping our lives, does it not seem logical to cultivate the ones that will set us on a journey to success?

We often talk about these healthy habits. How do we define them? If a habit must be considered healthy, it should benefit us physically, mentally and even emotionally. The habit must push us in the direction of progress.

In the beginning, forming such habits is hard as our life tends to take over. You need to consciously pursue a lifestyle that includes these habits in the beginning. It is only when you notice the benefits of these habits that they become your second skin.

This book talks about ten habits that have been proven to transform an individual's life. These habits not only ensure good health but also provide a sense of peace and fulfilment as they touch various levels of your being. The best part is that these habits are very simple. You don't have to worry about mastering them or becoming extraordinarily spiritual to feel the positive effects.

They are just some simple practices that we have forgotten in our life on the fast lane. Just stop and take a moment and allow yourself to shine with just a few simple inclusions in your routine.

Chapter 1: Hydrate

In many traditional sciences, water is referred to as the elixir of life. There is ample reason for this. To begin with, our body composition consists of 75% of water. That is nature's way of indicating to us the importance of water in sustaining life. There are many theories that you need to drink 8 glasses of water each day. While that is not exactly true, you need to make a conscious effort to consume as much water each day to maintain your health.

Water can be considered a nutrient. It is available as a liquid and also in several foods like cucumber and water melon. Try to include these foods in your diet to ensure that you replenish the water in your system continuously. We tend to lose a lot of water in the form of sweat and even when we breathe. This loss must be made up for.

When your body has enough water, bodily functions like transporting nutrients, producing hormones and enzymes and even simply maintaining the consistency of our blood becomes easy. This lets you function at the best of your abilities.

Water also detoxifies your body. Most toxins are soluble in water and are eliminated from the body when the water content is good enough. That means you will have great skin, healthy hair and a healthy body.

You can also control your weight with water. It is the best remedy for the extra calories that you might consume from time to time. Your muscles are energised and you are also able to process your thoughts better when your body has the required amount of water.

Remember, your body will give you cues when you need water. You may choose to drink water or even some juice or watery fruits. The only thing that you must not do is choose alcohol when your body gives you these cues. Alcohol has an effect that is entirely opposite to that of water. It tends to dehydrate your body and just replenishes all the toxins that you work so hard to get rid of. Keep water consumption high and alcohol consumption low and you will be on your way to great health and more powerful thoughts.

Chapter 2: Make Time for Yourself

Time is such a vital thing in our world today. It seems to be the one thing that nobody ever has enough of. It is almost like we are lost in the speed that everything around us seems to be moving at. So, it is very easy for us to give up on our dreams and just hang on to the very mundane and boring life that is actually quite draining.

The problem with all our thoughts today is that they seem to be detached from the person that we really are. What causes this? Maybe we do spend enough time with ourselves. As a result, we never pay attention to what we really want and are trying to constantly find an external locus of approval. No wonder our lives are so hard.

When we have a day off or even some time to ourselves, we tend to unwind before the television. However, too much TV can be something to think about. Today, the programmes are flooded with advertisements that tell us how much we need the things that are either completely unaffordable or simply of no use to us. But, we get caught up in the need to acquire these things to satisfy that external locus of appreciation that we just discussed.

What is the solution to this? It is very simple. All you need to do is introspect. Take some time off for yourself and think about the experiences that you have had in a day. What made you happy? What are the things that you would have done differently? It also pays to not think at all. Maybe unwind on your terrace or in a park close to your home. Staying close to nature is an excellent way to connect with yourself. That is when you are away from the expectations that people around you have set for you. So, you have the clarity to focus on your own needs.

It is during these moments of complete solitude that you will find answers to some questions that have really been bothering you. Whether it is a decision in your work place or a relationship that you are trying to manage, the real solution to any problem only lies within yourself. When you are sure of what you want, there is no confusion at all.

How would you ever find those solutions if you never made the time to be with yourself? So, make it a habit to take at least half an hour in a day to tune off from the world and tune into the innermost space of your being.

Chapter 3: Get Some Exercise

The benefits of exercise have been reiterated several times. We are bombarded with articles and programs that tell us how important exercise is. What most of them do not tell us is the effect that exercise has on our mental space. With exercise come many internal changes that improve our quality of life. Hence, this is a habit that you must cultivate.

Exercise benefits us physically, without a doubt. In addition to that, there are many chemicals like endorphins that are released when we exercise. These endorphins are also called happy hormones. They are able help us release stress, release inflammation and also reduce our resistance to insulin. In the process the brain is highly benefited. The survival of brain cells increases and there is a promotion of the growth of blood vessels in the brain as well. This is a significant advantage that will help us even in our aging process.

With these physiological changes comes the ability to control you moods and also sleep well. So, at the emotional level, too, you are sorted. The direct result of all this is that you are able to function better. Your cognition improves, which means that you are able to manage the different levels of your life, professional and personal. Studies have shown us that exercising helps boost our memory. With sustained practice of exercise for about one year or six months, researchers have measured a noticeable increase in the volume of certain brain regions that enhance our ability to process things.

How much exercise do you need to see these benefits? It is

good enough to engage in medium to high intensity workout for about one hour, thrice a week. Of course, you can also engage in regular physical activity on a daily basis. It could be a short walk around your block, cycling or even a session of dancing. All you need to do is give your heart something more to do for some time every day. The results will reflect in every area of your life.

Take every possible opportunity to go out and get some fresh air. It will clear your mind and will also help your body work to its best abilities. You will no longer have to be bothered by small ailments that compel you to pop a tablet every now and then. A body that is healthy is the reflection of a soul that is growing and blossoming.

Chapter 4: Clean Up Everyday

When you have clutter around you, your mind is in a mess, too. Try a simple exercise to understand what this means. Pick a task that you have to complete, preferably something work related. Now divide the task into two bits. Complete one bit in a room that is a mess. You must have clothes lying all over, piles of paper on the desk etc. Then, go to a clean space and finish the rest of your work. Note the time you take in both scenarios. Which one was faster?

Most people tend to work better in a clean space. You must make it a habit to clean something every day. This could even be something as simple as making your bed. When you are done with a cleaning process, it gives you that small sense of achievement that can carry you through the day feeling quite good about yourself.

Our need to be clean and organised, as many scientists have pointed it out, is almost an extension to the cleansing rituals that people have in religious ceremonies. Having some cleaning routine has actually helped many people deal with their low self-image. Research shows that when people carry any form of guilt, be it for unethical behaviour or even perceived bad behaviour, cleaning helps them deal with that.

Also, making your bed, cleaning out the garbage, doing the dishes etc. establish a moral and social standard. It alters the way people look at you. If you have a clean home and a clean working space at the office, you are perceived as a person who is in control of his actions. In a strange way, an organised person is often considered to be one step ahead of everybody else.

In a report entitled, "The Smell of Virtue", the details of an interesting experiment were noted down. In this experiment, volunteers were put in two rooms. One was clean scented and the other was called the baseline. Then, they were asked to participate in a trust game. There was a receiver and a sender. The sender would offer a certain amount of money that would be tripled and given to the sender. Now, the sender could split this money as he wanted and decide if he wanted to return any money at all. It was observed in this experiment that people in the clean scented room had sent back more money.

This experiment shows us that cleanliness in our environment does affect the way we think. In another part of this experiment, it was observed that people in the clean room were more likely to give money out as charity. So, it is alright to assume that our thoughts are cleansed when we clean the space around us.

Make it a point to at least make your bed every day. You will see that the clarity in your thought is significantly improved. You will be able to focus better. You are inclined towards having positive thoughts. This habit will stick with you for a long time when you practice it regularly as the benefits it has are many!

Chapter 5: Find a Hobby

They say that an idle mind is the workshop of the devil. This statement has been proved right on several occasions. You can even draw examples from your own life. It is likely that most of your unpleasant thoughts come to your when you are sitting before the TV or just lying on the bed with nothing to do.

When you are stuck in a routine, your spare time is like this time frame that you just want to skip. What do you do, just stay in bed all day? Weekends are subject to this type of idleness which can make you lethargic and unprepared when your week begins. This is probably why Monday blues are so common.

In order to prevent your mind from shutting off when you have some leisure, it is good to pursue a hobby. A hobby is clearly something that you enjoy. It could be something as simple as reading a book or even as complex as rock climbing. Most people have something that they absolutely love to do. If you are unsure of what that is, you could join a couple of classes or even join friends in their hobbies. When you find the hobby that can relax you and keep you interested, you will be able to lose yourself in it entirely.

It is true that hobbies make you more knowledgeable. Take coin collection for instance. You learn so much about various countries in the process. If it is a physically engaging hobby, you will learn about various aspects of fitness and nutrition. We usually become wiser with more knowledge.

Hobbies make great conversation starters. You will be able to find a social circle with interests similar to yours. When you are in a new social set up, you will also be able to break the ice easily because you are now equipped with a lot more information in general. This information will also favour you in your profession as you will be able to add value to the tasks that you are required to execute.

Many times, people are lucky to find a lucrative breakthrough in their hobbies. If you are one of them, you will be able to do something that you absolutely love for a living. This prospect itself is motivation enough for you to look for a hobby and make it a habit to dedicate some time every day or month towards that hobby.

Chapter 6: Positive Self-Talk

Have you ever paid any attention to the conversation that you normally have with yourself? If you haven't, try it. Most often, our talks with ourselves include embarrassing incidents, heartbreaks, problems, financial struggles, loss and displeasure. We seldom talk to ourselves. We only tend to brood. Now, this brooding is facilitated by the social media which projects everyone else's life as perfect. When you are constantly bashing yourself up, do you think that innovation and creativity have any room? You don't like your own opinions and ideas. So, you will never be able to create anything original.

If you look at the trend in the world today, originality is rare. People are able to improvise on existing ideas but that spark of madness seems to be missing. This issue may be solved if people are able to love themselves more. Then, the need to impress the world will stop. When you start doing things for yourself, you will find it a lot more interesting. You will also be able to get better results as you are being completely honest to what you really believe in.

If you are wondering how one can know if he loves himself or not, the answer is quite simple. It really does not matter. Make it a point to include "being kind to yourself" in your list of habits. Each morning, wake up and remind yourself that you are alive for a reason. There is always something great that you can look forward to. Look at yourself in the mirror and point out one good thing that you see.

If you are able to vocalise this affection for yourself, the results are faster. Tell yourself that you are beautiful and that you deserve to have all your dreams fulfilled. There is a strange sense of assurance when you do this. If you are someone who loves to work out, you may have noticed that when you are in that last, tiring set, just telling yourself that you can push harder actually helps. If this works in the gym, there is no reason why it should not work in real life. Make it a habit to say something positive and kind to yourself every day, whenever possible.

Chapter 7: Kindness is Habitual

In the German legend of Faust, the protagonist is extremely unhappy with his life. He decides to make a pact with the devil for one moment of pure happiness in exchange for eternal damnation. He comes across a man who is crippled in an accident. Faust offers to help the man and soon finds himself helping more people. The legend of Faust, however, has a tragic ending when his acts of corruption ultimately lead him to hell.

In our lives, we are constantly looking for solace and peace. We try to accomplish this through our achievements in our profession and in our perceived sense of luxury. But, real and complete happiness was never really that hard. It was always simple. If you see the happiest people in the world, you will notice one similar quality in all of them. They are all selfless. They find joy in doing something for another person, no matter how small the act is. Had Faust found the pleasure of helping people in the first place, he would never be condemned to eternal misery.

If you are in the pursuit of happiness, develop one simple habit. Try to do one nice thing for someone else every day. You could buy a sandwich for a homeless person, lend an umbrella to someone who needs it or just listen to someone who really wants another person to talk to. Today, most people associate kindness with charity. If you have the means to reduce the monetary problems in someone's life, you may do it. But if you are not up to it yet, there is so much more that you can do to feel the joy of helping another person.

When you experience the genuine gratitude of another person, you will find that nothing else matters as much. The joy that you get when you are responsible for the smile on another person's face is irreplaceable. When you make this a habit, you will notice that your own insecurities, your lack of contentment and your final purpose will change significantly. The worldly pleasures, as important as they are, will not be the underlying factor for everything that you do.

In a sense, when you are able to help another person, you are truly liberated. This freedom will reflect on your entire life.

Chapter 8: Forget your Failures

Our past generally determines the way we think about our lives. If we were unable to succeed at one thing in our lives, we develop a mental block towards it for life. Thankfully, there are stories of legends that have turned failure into the stepping stone of their success stories. Instead of dwelling on their failures, they were able to take the rejection or that low point in their life as a challenge. They drew inspiration from their failures and went on to achieve greatness.

Let us take the story of the Beatles, for instance. They were rejected by Decca records who said that "The Beatles have no future in the music industry." This is considered the biggest blunder in the history of the music industry. We all know what a sensation the Beatles began. In fact, the rejected audition tape was auctioned for a fortune a few years later. Would the Beatles have ever succeeded if they had been disheartened by these comments? This occured in a time when the verdict of Decca Records was considered the final word in deciding the future of a music group.

If you have experienced failure, be thankful. There is no better teacher than failure. Try to understand what went wrong and tell yourself, "I will get this right the next time." One failure does not seal your fate. Unless you are able to understand this, there is no way you will be able to grow and succeed in your endeavours. Once you have failed at something, there is not much you can do about that. You cannot go over that incident in your head several times, feeling miserable about it.

The wiser thing to do would be to prepare yourself for the next step. What can you do in the future to avoid these mistakes? When you do this, you will also notice that the quality of the effort that you put in is better. So, the results are bound to be better.

While it is important not to dwell on failures, it is also not the best idea to cling to your achievements. Allow your achievements to motivate you in trying times. But, make sure that they do not limit you. Use your achievements as proof that you can do more. If you were able to achieve that, you are capable of doing better.

Consciously remind yourself to forget about the past and look forward to the brighter and more promising future. That is the only way to progress in any field of work or even in your personal space.

Chapter 9: Find Good Company

Epictetus said, "The key is to keep company only with people who uplift you, whose presence calls forth your best." In these simple words, he has provided the ultimate solution to problems like the lack of motivation.

The people who are around you must be genuine. There is no point being around people who will put you on a pedestal without reason. These are the people who do not really care about your growth. You see, when we are underachieving or when we are at fault, we know it at a very subconscious level. When you are with real friends and people who are truly concerned about helping you get better, you will notice that they are encouraging without making everything sound like a fairy tale. They will give you solutions that are practical. And, when necessary, they will be tough on you and push you towards success.

It is also dangerous to be around people who are constantly holding you back. We all fall into the company of certain people who tend to be condescending. They will make it a point to be ominous about everything that you do. These people should be kept at bay. Their opinions can, most of the times, shake even your strongest beliefs.

It is good to be around people who are similar to you. They must be willing to work hard. They should have had good life experiences that have given them valuable lessons that they will be able to share with you. They should be able to add value to what you are already doing in order to promote your chances of reaching your goals faster. These people can be your colleagues, your friends and, certainly, your family.

There is no need to look at everyone with a sense of judgment. However, when you find the right people be sensitive to the vibes that you get from them. If people are able to make you feel secure and confident, then you are probably in the right company. You should be able to speak your mind without worrying about what they may think. That is when you are really putting yourself in a situation that enables growth.

If, even for a moment, you feel the need to pretend to be someone else, you need to leave that company immediately. When you are not even yourself, how will you ever get any help there to get to the goals that you have set? Make sure that you are at ease when you are with your peers. If you are not, then you are definitely not in progressive company.

The law of attraction says that you are most likely to attract people who think and feel like you. Therefore, if you trying to find the right company, make it a habit to be the person you really are.

Chapter 10: Compliment Strangers

"Do unto others as you would have them do unto you." This statement is one of the most powerful ones that exist. If you want people to look at you and appreciate you, you must start doing so yourself. It is very simple to compliment people whom we know well. However, the real challenge comes when you are trying to find something positive in a complete stranger. If you try to compliment a stranger every day, you will be surprised at how different your thought process becomes. Since it is a habit that you are trying to form, you will consciously look for the beauty around you. Now, if that isn't refreshing, I do not know what else is.

With strangers, a compliment comes at the risk of being perceived as creepy, especially if you are complimenting someone of the opposite gender. To make things more social, there are a few rules of thumb rules that you can follow. Maintain eye contact. When you do this, your intentions are seldom questioned. Keep a friendly gaze and tell the person what you find nice about them.

Make sure that your compliments are not limited to the physical appearance. Yes, you may love someone's hairdo or dress. Then, be vocal about that. Try to compliment something that they are doing. For instance, if you are sitting in a busy coffee shop, tell the waiter, "I think you are doing such a great job serving so many people at once." This will undoubtedly make that person's day. If you saw someone share some food with a homeless person a simple, "What you did was really sweet," is the best compliment you can give that person.

Complimenting strangers becomes a habit with practice. It is not easy. So, you need to do it more often. Leave you house every day with the goal of complimenting at least one stranger. As you get used to it, you will become more comfortable doing it. This habit really helps you in other ways. You will never experience nerves when you are speaking to strangers. This ability to speak to strangers will give you a renewed sense of confidence. You will also feel really good about yourself because you were able to make another person happy, even if it was for a moment.

Remember that everyone around us is looking for some appreciation. Wouldn't you like it if someone pointed out something nice about you? Just go ahead and do this for someone else, too. You just need to be genuine. Don't expect them to say something in return. You may even get snubbed sometimes. It's alright, don't let that dishearten you. That person probably had a terrible day at work. Continue your efforts to be nice and you will see how everything just seems to be in place and perfect. Beauty lies in the eye of the beholder. All you need to do is train your eyes on a regular basis.

Conclusion

These habits are no doubt, extremely simple. Initially, you could even make a to do list of healthy habits. People are often overwhelmed when they hear the phrase, "form positive habits." Positive habits include things like stopping junk food, always being nice or letting go of bad habits. Therefore, it seems like a stretch to have positive habits in your life. However, habits are a lot simpler than that.

They have tremendous power over us and can determine the way our lives shape out. But, let's face it, nobody can be 100% perfect. You cannot be a person with only good habits. What you can be is a person willing to change the bad habits for the better. Even the idea that you want to make your life better will push you in the right direction.

In order to cultivate good habits, start with a plan. Draw a thirty day chart that focuses on one or two of the habits mentioned in this book. Make it a point to execute them. When you do, make a note of how you feel when you pursue a certain habit. At the end of thirty days, go through these notes and you will realise why these habits were worth all the effort. It is said that anything you do repeatedly, on a daily basis for 30 to 45 days becomes a habit and stays with you. Once you have formed some habits, use the same methods to cultivate new ones.

When you have tasted the effects of all the above habits in your life, you will not want to let go. You will see a change in your personal life, in your profession and also on a very individual level. It is possible to feel more content with the way your life is shaping up by developing these positive habits.

I hope that you find this book helpful. Making a transition into a more meaningful life is something that we all want. The only thing that is stopping us is our routines and our lack of sensitivity towards the world that we live in. Our habits have the ability to really change our perspective on various things.

To quote Aristotle:

"We are what we do repeatedly. Excellence, then, is not an act, but a habit."